"Alex Attewell has captured the thrilling essence and (Nightingale's message that re-awakens nurses and nur their own calling. Re-connecting to their true heritage and professional roots empowers nurses in health advocacy for creating a healthy world—local to global."

–Barbara Dossey, PhD, RN, AHN-BC, FAAN
International Co-director, Nightingale Initiative for Global Health
Ottawa, Ontario, Canada, and Arlington, Virginia
Author, Florence Nightingale: Mystic, Visionary, Healer and
Holistic Nursing: A Handbook for Practice

"Alex Attewell's new book, *Illuminating Florence: Finding Nightingale's Legacy in Your Practice*, is a wonderful gem of a reference for the practicing nurse. Capturing some of Nightingale's most inspiring insights, Attewell reveals his extensive knowledge of nursing's icon and her relevance today. The book is lovingly illustrated with historical photos of Florence throughout her life, coupled with modern images of nursing. This book would make a great gift for a colleague or graduating student."

–Abby Heydman, PhD, RN
Professor and Academic Vice President Emerita
Samuel Merritt University

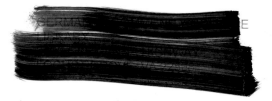

"There is much myth and mystery that swirls around Florence Nightingale. However, she was a prolific writer of letters, books, official documents, and private notes that reveal her innermost thoughts. Alex Attewell has been able to bring this wealth of material into a useful volume for the reader to easily and accurately access Nightingale's perception of the potential of nursing and the importance that the individual nurse brings to the profession."

–Louise Selanders, EdD, RN, FAAN
Director of Master Programs
College of Nursing
Michigan State University

"In an amazingly economical way, Attewell uses pithy prose and skillfully selected quotes to capture the essence of Florence Nightingale's prodigious contributions to the profession of nursing. Through the artful juxtaposition of original text, historical photographs, and commentary, he focuses the Nightingale lens on a more accurate and magnanimous depiction that will inspire generations of nurses to come. This concise yet powerful book is a tour de force in Nightingale scholarship."

–Joan M. Pryor McCann, PhD, RN, CNS, CNL
Professor of Nursing
Director of Undergraduate Studies
Director of the Clinical Nurse Leader Program
Otterbein University

"Attewell has written an inspirational book that captures the timelessness of Florence Nightingale's legacy on nursing's contribution to health of humankind. Her call to action and reminder that only people can act are relevant today. Florence Nightingale was a leader who continues to make a difference. Attewell fills the book with her quotes that guide our practice today. A must-read!"

–*Marilyn P. Chow, RN, DNSc, FAAN*
Vice President
National Patient Care Services
Kaiser Permanente

"An attractive and stylish book on Florence Nightingale and her relevance for nurses today. Here at last is an accessible guide to the ways in which Nightingale's nursing doctrines still speak to us, more than a century after her death."

–*Mark Bostridge*
Author of Florence Nightingale: The Woman and Her Legend

"*Illuminating Florence* is a helpful addition to works on Florence Nightingale. By highlighting her achievements in leadership and her firmly held beliefs that health care is as much about maintaining health and wellbeing as it is about treating disease, this book puts her work in a modern-day context. The selection of timeless quotes serves to underpin the relevance and qualities of Florence Nightingale to contemporary nursing practice and a culture of continuous improvement in the quality of care."

–Professor Elizabeth Robb, (Hons D Univ), MA, BA (Hons), RN, RM, ADM, PGCEA
Chief Executive, Florence Nightingale Foundation

"After inspiring so many, including me—her cousin—to study Florence Nightingale, her life, aspirations, and vision, Alex has now written his own thought-provoking assessment of the many aspects of this remarkable lady. It has been my privilege to have been associated with him and to have benefitted from his wide knowledge."

–Margaret Povey
First cousin (twice removed) of Florence Nightingale
(her grandfather, General Sir Lothian Nicholson, was a first cousin of
Florence Nightingale and served with the Royal Engineers in the Crimean War)
St. Thomas Hospital Nightingale Nurse, 1954 (Retired)

"A timely and remarkable resource for every nurse's library!"

–Diane Mancino, EdD, RN, CAE, FAAN

illuminating
florence

finding nightingale's legacy in your practice

Alex Attewell, MBA, BA, AMA

Sigma Theta Tau International
Honor Society of Nursing®

The Honor Society of Nursing, Sigma Theta Tau International (STTI) is a nonprofit organization whose mission is to support the learning, knowledge, and professional development of nurses committed to making a difference in health worldwide. Founded in 1922, STTI has 125,000 members in 90 countries. Members include practicing nurses, instructors, researchers, policymakers, entrepreneurs and others. STTI's 486 chapters are located throughout Australia, Botswana, Brazil, Canada, Colombia, England, Ghana, Hong Kong, Japan, Kenya, Malawi, Mexico, Netherlands, Pakistan, Singapore, South Africa, South Korea, Swaziland, Sweden, Taiwan, Tanzania, the United States, and Wales. More information about STTI can be found online at www.nursingsociety.org

Sigma Theta Tau International
550 West North Street
Indianapolis, IN, USA 46202

To order additional books, buy in bulk, or order for corporate use, contact Nursing Knowledge International at 888.NKI.4YOU (888.654.4968/US and Canada) or +1.317.634.8171 (outside US and Canada).

To request a review copy for course adoption, e-mail solutions@nursingknowledge.org or call 888.NKI.4YOU (888.654.4968/US and Canada) or +1.317.634.8171 (outside US and Canada).

To request author information, or for speaker or other media requests, contact Rachael McLaughlin of the Honor Society of Nursing, Sigma Theta Tau International at 888.634.7575 (US and Canada) or +1.317.634.8171 (outside US and Canada).

Library of Congress Cataloging-in-Publication Data

Attewell, Alex.

Illuminating Florence : finding Nightingale's legacy in your practice / Alex Attewell.

p. ; cm.

Includes bibliographical references.

ISBN 978-1-937554-50-7 (alk. paper) -- ISBN 978-1-937554-51-4 (EPUB) --
ISBN 978-1-937554-52-1 (PDF) -- ISBN 978-1-937554-53-8 (MOBI)

I. Sigma Theta Tau International. II. Title.

[DNLM: 1. Nightingale, Florence, 1820-1910. 2. Nurses--Biography. 3. History of Nursing--
Biography. 4. History, 19th Century--Biography. 5. History, 20th Century--Biography. 6.
Nursing--Biography. WZ 100]

LC classification not assigned

610.73092--dc23

[B]

2012019154

Publisher: Renee Wilmeth

Acquisitions Editor: Emily Hatch

Cover & Interior Designer: Rebecca Batchelor

Editorial Coordinator: Paula Jeffers

Principal Book Editor: Carla Hall

Proofreader: Jane Palmer

Editor's Note: Nightingale's words are reproduced with occasional and minor editing of spelling.

All image rights as credited in the Table of Images beginning on page 79.

ISBN: 9781937554507

First Printing, 2012

Dedication

For my wife, Sofía, and my nan, Hilda, the first nurse in my life.

Acknowledgements

I am grateful to all the librarians and archivists who have helped me with source material, particularly at the Wellcome Trust and the British Library. My heartfelt thanks to all my former colleagues—the staff, volunteers, and associates of the Florence Nightingale Museum in London—for everything I have learned about nursing from them and for their practical help with research. It was an immense privilege to be involved with the preservation of the Nightingale heritage, for which I acknowledge the museum trustees. I owe a debt to many historians of Florence Nightingale whom I have had the pleasure to know over the years. I particularly thank my friend, Professor Louise Selanders at Michigan State University, for some last-minute help with sources. I would like to express my grateful thanks to my colleagues at Sigma Theta Tau International for their support on this project, particularly to Emily Hatch.

The copyright of Florence Nightingale's writings rests with the Henry Bonham-Carter Will Trust. I am very grateful to Radcliffes Solicitors Limited, which administers the Henry Bonham-Carter Will Trust, for permission to publish the Florence Nightingale quotes in this book.

About the Author

Alex Attewell, MBA, BA, AMA, is a history honors graduate of the University of Bristol. He qualified as a social history curator through Leicester University and the Museums Association in 1992, and he completed his MBA through Kingston University in 2004. Attewell began his 18-year career with the Florence Nightingale Museum in London in 1989, serving as the assistant curator, curator, and then director. Under his direction, the museum grew as an educational and research center with a range of exhibitions and educational services for nurses and school children. He has curated and managed exhibitions, and he continues to lecture and broadcast on Florence Nightingale in the United Kingdom, Europe, and the United States. The Florence Nightingale Museum won various awards and accolades under his management, including recognition as one of the Top 10 United Kingdom Small Museums (*The Independent*) and Best Exhibition in London (*The Times*). Named an honorary member of the Honor Society of Nursing, Sigma Theta Tau International in 2001, Attewell now resides in Quintana Roo, Mexico. In addition to lecturing about Florence Nightingale and conducting Nightingale-related historical tours, Attewell operates a Spanish-English translation business and continues to write.

References

Attewell, A. (2010). Florence Nightingale's relevance to nurses. *Journal of Holistic Nursing, 28*(1), 101-106.

Bostridge, M. (2008). *Florence Nightingale: The making of an icon,* New York, NY: Farrar, Straus and Giroux.

Carrier-Walker, L. (2009). *Notes on nursing: A guide for today's caregivers.* Edinburgh; Scotland: Elsevier/Baillière Tindall.

Dossey, B. (2010). *Florence Nightingale: Mystic, visionary, healer.* Philadelphia, PA: F. A. Davis Company.

Dossey, B., Selanders, L. C., Beck, D.-M., & Attewell, A. (2004). *Florence Nightingale today: Healing, leadership, global action.* Silver Spring, MD: American Nurses Association.

Nightingale, F. (1863). *Notes on hospitals.* London, UK: Longman, Green, Longman, Roberts, & Green. (Note: the original reference is given as there is no reprint currently available.)

Rafferty, A.-M., & Wall, R. (2010). An icon or iconoclast. In S. Nelson & A.-M. Rafferty (Eds.), *Notes on Nightingale.* Ithaca, NY: Cornell University Press.

Selanders, L. C. (1993). *Florence Nightingale: An environmental adaptation theory.* Newbury Park, CA: Sage Publications.

Skretkowicz, V. (Ed.). (2010). *Notes on nursing: What it is and what it is not & notes on nursing for the labouring classes.* New York, NY: Springer Publishing Company.

Small, H. (1999). *Florence Nightingale: Avenging angel.* New York, NY: St. Martin's Press.

Additional Reading

The most readily accessible versions of most of Florence Nightingale's writings are in the Collected Works of Florence Nightingale, Lynn McDonald (Ed.), published by the Wilfrid Laurier University Press, Waterloo, ON, Canada. The most relevant volumes are (1) *Life and Family,* (2) *Spiritual Journey,* (5) *Society and Politics,* (6) *Public Health Care,* (8) *Women,* (9) *Florence Nightingale on Health in India,* (11) *Florence Nightingale's Suggestions for Thought,* (12) *The Nightingale School,* (13) *Extending Nursing, and (15) Wars and the War Office.*

Table of Contents

Foreword

I am delighted to write the foreword to *Illuminating Florence: Finding Nightingale's Legacy in Your Practice,* what you might call a pocket guide to Florence Nightingale's relevance to today's nurses.

In 2009, the International Council of Nurses and its sister foundation, the Florence Nightingale International Foundation, produced a modern version of Nightingale's *Notes on Nursing*, which provided up-to-date nursing knowledge while retaining Nightingale's key themes and essence.

Similarly, *Illuminating Florence* shows us that there is much that we can still learn from Nightingale today. By providing quotes and giving the historical background to these "sound bites," Alex Attewell examines Nightingale's words and work, showing how her legacy continues to contribute to nursing knowledge, nursing organization, and nursing education.

There is no doubt that Florence Nightingale's influence on nursing continues more than 100 years after her death. She personifies many of the important ideas that are crucial to nursing today: values, vision, and voice. Many of the quotes selected for this book bring to mind issues that we are facing today: for example, "*causes which we could so well remove*" (lifestyle choices that are the cause of many non-communicable diseases), the need for "*important statistics,*" or the use of evidence-based approaches to nursing services.

As former director of the Florence Nightingale Museum in London, Attewell's intimate knowledge and tremendous respect for Florence Nightingale are evident. Through her quotes, historical and modern photographs, other images, and reproductions of parts of her letters, Attewell's book highlights her vision of nursing, her contribution to nursing management, her view of leadership, her definition of patient care, and how her legacy lives on.

–David C. Benton
Chief Executive Officer
International Council of Nurses

Introduction

As astounding as it might be, modern nursing can still learn from nursing in the 19th century. As well as being a nursing icon, Florence Nightingale was remarkably wise and forward thinking, and had a lot of common sense. Her insights, comments, and recommendations are well over 100 years old and yet they remain fresh, powerful, and of direct relevance to clinical nursing practice today; further, her principles continue to have an important bearing on nursing management and leadership.

This book features a selection of timeless quotes taken from Nightingale's writings. If she were alive today, I hope she would appreciate the *efficiency* of this selection. *Efficiency* is, in fact, a word usage she pioneered in nursing (in her day, the only other people who tended to use it were engineers). The length of this book does not even come close to one thousandth of the volume of her literary output. It aims to make a virtue of brevity, highlighting the most relevant points among a huge mass of information, as Nightingale herself was well known for doing. And, it illuminates the relevance of these words through the use of historical and modern imagery, making her messages as beautiful as they are powerful and relevant.

Around 20 years ago, I observed a nurse viewing the exhibit at the Florence Nightingale Museum, reading aloud a Nightingale quote and commenting—I'm paraphrasing here—"That's exactly what we mean by holistic care today!" It is interesting that the word "holism" did not feature in the exhibit, but it was clearly what Nightingale was talking about more than 150 years ago! You create the relevance as a nurse by engaging with the past from your modern perspective.

The quotes here have all been selected for their interest to nurses and have been organized with commentaries to show some development in Florence's thoughts around five themes—Vision, Management, Leadership, Theory, and Legacy—but I have intentionally not spelled out what the relevance might be or should be for you, in the hope that you will use the book as a means of reflecting on your own practice as a nurse.

The first and last chapters, on Vision and Legacy, respectively, are like the bookends and bracket Florence Nightingale's thinking on Management, Leadership, and Theory (of nursing practice). These first and last chapters have a more personal feel, representing the spiritual and intellectual motivations that brought her into nursing and then, finally, the legacy she left to nurses and nursing.

For too long, Florence Nightingale has been thought of just as the "lady with the lamp," a heroic figure from nursing's past. I hope that after reading *Illuminating Florence*, you will reconsider her legacy in regard to your own contemporary practice and ask yourself the critical questions: Is her legacy relevant to your practice? If so, how can her experiences help you to re-imagine the role of nurses in the light of today's health care challenges?

–Alex Attewell

1

vision

Florence Nightingale in the garden at Embley Park, 1858. While the story of the young Florence hearing the voice of God in the garden at

In her early years, Florence Nightingale continually reflected on her purpose in life and the meaning of disease and suffering. As a young woman, Nightingale had a strong sense of her vocation as a nurse, which perhaps she needed if ever she was to overcome the prejudices against nursing among her wealthy and educated class. Such was the weight of conventional expectation that when she eventually broke through, she became one of only a few educated women of her generation with a role in the public sphere. She finally freed herself from family constraints to become involved in nursing at the age of 31, and so perhaps it is not surprising that her early years of inactivity gave her an impatience for action. Hers was an intensely practical vision.

After her work during the Crimean War (1854-56), Florence Nightingale was in a unique position to address the reform of army health care and then the organization of nursing education in civil hospitals. Subsequently, she promoted preventive measures which included healthier army barracks in peacetime and measures to address alcoholism. Her Crimean fame and the connections she gathered in the process of army reform opened up

Embley is probably apocryphal, it is undoubtedly true that the time she spent there in reflection was vital to the development of her vision.

possibilities for the application of her vision that she had barely dreamed of. The fourth quote on page 13, about the inadequacy of good intentions gives a good indication of how finely tuned her vision was for the opportunities and challenges she faced.

As a reformer, Nightingale's vision led her to look to the ideal, which she tempered with political reality. While engaged in the cut and thrust of reforms, she rarely expressed a clear vision of the future; it would have presented a clear target for those who opposed her schemes. In her later years, as she moved beyond involvement in government administration, she expressed a wider-ranging vision for the future of nursing that emphasized wellness. The final quote on page 16 is from her paper "Sick Nursing and Health Nursing," which was read out at the World's Columbian Exposition of 1893. It contains Nightingale's most significant visionary statements about the nurse's role in the prevention of disease and maintaining people in good health. It repeats an assertion made by Nightingale many times over the years—that hospitals are an "intermediate stage of civilization," as she believed that it would ultimately be cheaper to maintain people in health than to treat disease.

It is interesting that Nightingale did not value writing unless it brought practical benefits. If she were reading these words now, her response might go along these lines: "How does this writing link with the Millennium Development Goals? Do people still listen when they hear my name? Why not point out that I was saying precisely the same things about saving lives through clean water, health education, and the improvement of children's health more than 100 years ago. Let's see some real progress now."

Nightingale's vision has an all-embracing quality, from the spiritual and personal to the global dimensions. Her relevance is not in precisely the brand of Christian spirituality she believed in, but rather the value of being spiritual, having inner belief and commitment which link the dimensions of a nurse's work and personal life.

the hospital of
your dreams

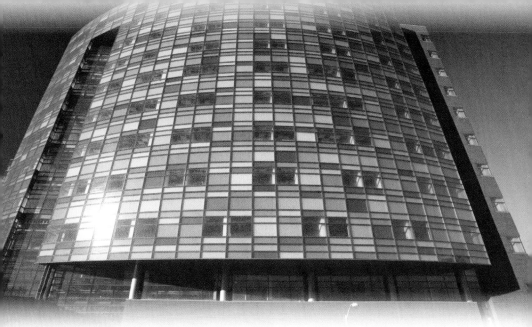

"*My daydreams were all of hospitals and I visited them whenever I could. I never communicated it to anyone—it would have been laughed at—but I thought God called me to serve Him in that way.*"

(Curriculum Vitae, 1850)

7

stop talking and start doing

"I think one's feelings waste themselves in words; they ought all to be distilled into actions which bring results."

(Letter to her friend Mary Clarke, 1844)

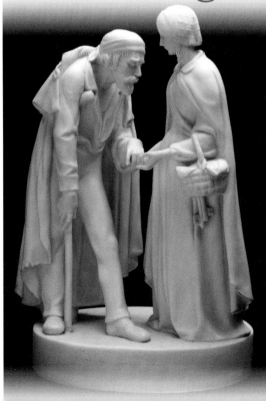

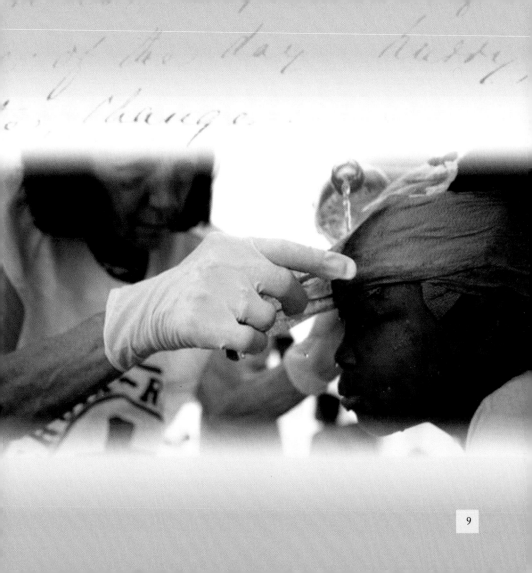

how do we respond to today's health challenges?

"It did strike me as odd, sometimes, that we should pray to be delivered 'from plague, pestilence, and famine,' when all the common sewers ran into the Thames, and fevers haunted undrained land, and the districts which cholera would visit could be pointed out. I thought that cholera came that we might remove these causes, not pray that God would remove the cholera."

(Suggestions for Thought, 1860)

good intentions are not enough

12

"*The kingdom of heaven is within, but we must also make it without. … Good intentions are supposed enough, yet blunders, organized blunders, do so much more mischief than crimes. … Indeed, organized carelessness is more hurtful even than actual sin, as every day we have cause to find out.*" *(Fraser's Magazine, 1873)*

learning through doing

"*Book learning is useful only to render the practical health of the health workshop intelligent, so that every stroke of work done there should be felt to be an illustration of what has been learnt elsewhere, a driving home, by an experience not to be forgotten, what has been gained by knowledge too easily forgotten. Look for the ideal, but put it into the actual.*" (Sick Nursing and Health Nursing, 1893)

management

The bust of Florence Nightingale by Sir John Steell, 1862, was sculpted in a classical style usually reserved for male members of the establishment. It was commissioned by the ordinary soldiers of the British army who were nursed back to health by Nightingale and her colleagues

Understanding Florence Nightingale's contribution to management as a unified whole is a challenge. It embraces the 3 years of intense hands-on work as a nurse manager—including her time in the Crimean War—and the many subsequent years of writing, campaigning, and expert consultancy linked to that period. In focusing on her contribution to management from a nursing perspective, we must draw together her work on the management of nurses, nurse education, statistical work, hospital planning, and social reform. The quotes appearing in this section are about health-improvement management.

The "Diagram of the Causes of Mortality in the Army in the East" on page 20 had only one purpose: to show that the majority of British army deaths in the Crimean War were preventable. The area of the blue wedges in this polar-area diagram represents deaths from preventable or mitigable diseases, such as dysentery and typhoid. The area of the red wedges represents deaths from wounds, and the area of the black wedges represents deaths from other causes. It first appeared in Nightingale's 1858 report to the government, which may be regarded as a groundbreaking clinical audit.

during the Crimean War. The loyal support of her former patients gave her the authority she needed for her campaign to improve army health management.

Persistence was one of Florence Nightingale's characteristics as a manager, and this is well represented by an often-repeated phrase she scribbled as a personal reminder: "Reports are not self-executive." After the Crimean War, she vowed that the blunders that had led to so many preventable deaths from disease should never be repeated and wrote numerous reports to government leaders with practical recommendations. She often oversaw the implementation of her reports in minute detail, but equally she found that the strategic and controlled disclosure of an unpublished report could achieve the desired results.

Nightingale learned about complex organizational processes through her management experience in the Crimean War, and her groundbreaking third edition of *Notes on Hospitals*, 1863, evolved from her government reports on the mismanagement of military hospitals in the war. She had a hospital-outcome nomenclature endorsed by an international statistical congress. She designed forms, and her design of a hospital-benchmarking scheme was trialed in London in the 1860s. Unfortunately, her ideas were so advanced that it was more than 100 years until her benchmarking ideas were again put into practice.

Before Nightingale established her clinical nurse training at St Thomas' Hospital in London in 1860, she set up a framework for military nurse training that did not go ahead exactly as planned, but her writing shows that she conceived of nurse training in the context of overall health care improvement. The formal letter to the nurses, beginning on page 71, shows how she imbued nursing with the idea of continual progress and development. She wrote 13 such letters to the probationer and qualified nurses at St. Thomas', and continuous learning is one of the central themes.

Much of Nightingale's writing on hospital design focuses on sanitation because it was the central health issue of her day, as she herself had demonstrated with her Crimean statistics. As sanitation has since been standardized in the developed world, the results of Nightingale's research are less relevant today, but the relevance is in her evidence-based methods and principles. Her quote on cost and fitness for purpose exemplifies this.

statistics

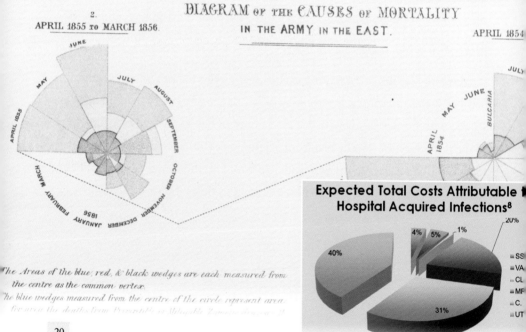

2.
APRIL 1855 to MARCH 1856.

DIAGRAM of the CAUSES of MORTALITY
IN THE ARMY IN THE EAST.

APRIL 1854

The Areas of the blue, red, & black wedges are each measured from
the centre as the common vertex.
The blue wedges measured from the centre of the circle represent area

Expected Total Costs Attributable to Hospital Acquired Infections[8]

"Improved statistics would tell us more of the relative value of particular operations and modes of treatment than we have any means of ascertaining at present ... and the truth thus ascertained would enable us to save life and suffering, and to improve the treatment and management of the sick. ... It need hardly be pointed out of what great practical value these and similar results would become ... hospitals might be compared with hospitals and wards with wards. The whole question of hospital economics as influenced by diets, medicines, comforts, could be brought under examination and discussion."
(Notes on Hospitals, 1863)

data is
passive;
only
people
can act

MORTALITY

OF THE

BRITISH ARMY,

AT HOME, AT HOME AND ABROAD, AND DURING THE RUSSIAN WAR,

AS COMPARED WITH THE

MORTALITY OF THE CIVIL POPULATION IN ENGLAND.

Illustrated by Tables and Diagrams.

Reprinted from the Report of the Royal Commission appointed to enquire into the Regulations affecting the Sanitary State of the Army.

LONDON:

PRINTED BY HARRISON AND SONS, ST. MARTIN'S LANE.

1858.

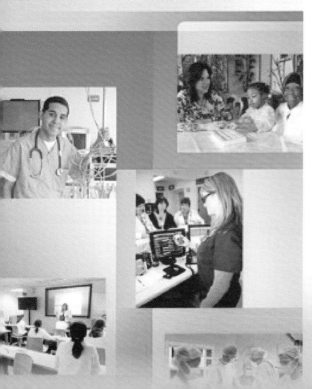

he Future of Nursing:

EADING CHANGE, ADVANCING HEALTH

"*Reports are not self-executive.*"

(Note of July 1858, repeated continually over the following years.)

the role of nursing in improving health care

Nurses sent to the Military Hospitals in the East. *Engaged by Miss Nightingale Oct. 1854.*

Country, and Condition.	Age.	Residence.	Where Trained or Practised.	Guarantees and Character.	When and Where sent.	Remarks.
... Florence ...tingale ...intendent of Nurses.		7 Lea Hurst Matlock 2 Embley Romsey.			Scutari Oct. 23 1854	Returned Aug...
...ebecca Lawfield		St John's House Queen's Sqt. Westminster	St John's House	do	Scutari Oct. 23. General Hospital.	Genl. Hospl. became R. Catholic. Returned with detachment...
...beth Drake.		St John's House	St John's House	do	Scutari Oct. 23 General Hosp.	died at Balaclava Aug. 10th 5 a most exemplary & excellent Nurse
... Higgins		St John's House	St John's House	do	Scutari Oct. 23	Sent home Jan... incompetent

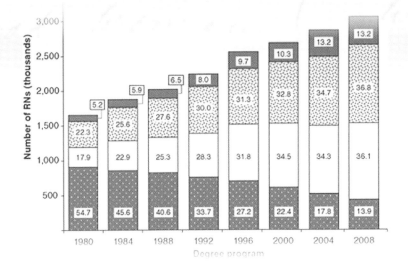

Number of RNs (thousands)

	1980	1984	1988	1992	1996	2000	2004	2008
	5.2	5.9	6.5	8.0	9.7	10.3	13.2	13.2
	22.3	25.6	27.6	30.0	31.3	32.8	34.7	36.8
	17.9	22.9	25.3	28.3	31.8	34.5	34.3	36.1
	54.7	45.6	40.6	33.7	27.2	22.4	17.8	13.9

Degree program

"*The main object I conceive to be, to improve hospitals, by improving hospital-nursing; and to do this by improving, or contributing towards the improvement, of the class of hospital-nurses, whether nurses or head nurses.*"

(Subsidiary Notes as to the Introduction of Female Nursing Into Military Hospitals in Peace and in War, 1858)

the design
of hospitals

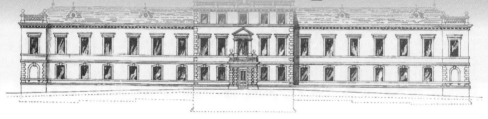

SOUTH ELEVATION.

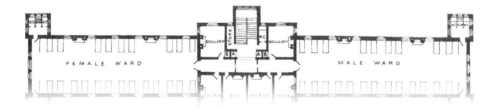

FEMALE WARD   SCULLERY STORE W.C SCULLERY   MALE WARD

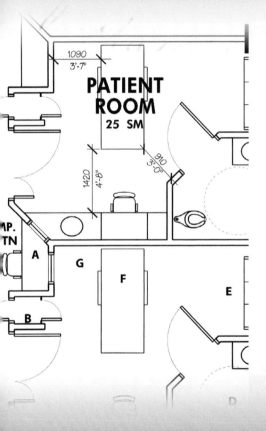

"It should never be forgotten that the first thing to be considered is what is best for the sick, not what may appear to be cheapest. … The very first condition to be sought in planning a building is, that it should be fit for its purpose."

(Notes on Hospitals, 1863)

3

leadership

Florence Nightingale in the blue room at Claydon House, the home of
Sir Harry Verney, her brother-in-law and a member of the British
parliament for many years. Verney gave political support for many of

Florence Nightingale was one of nursing's greatest leaders, and her thinking on leadership is insightful and relevant. The first two quotes in this chapter give biographical insight into Nightingale as a leader. The first, written before her life's great opportunities arose, highlights the importance of vision to leadership. It is undoubtedly true that Nightingale was able to grasp her principal leadership opportunity because she already had a sense of vocation and had reflected amply on what she might contribute. The second quote is about Nightingale's fearless sense of responsibility, one of her key personal traits as a leader. One of her greatest criticisms at Scutari was the poor leadership shown in the crisis months, when none of her colleagues were willing to take responsibility. For her part, Nightingale cut red tape, and at the risk of personal unpopularity, went over the heads of commanders to obtain critical supplies for her hospitals.

The third quote gives one very small example of how she chose to exercise her leadership. In her post-Crimean role as a nurse leader, Nightingale chose to champion the health of the people of India. (She supported many other causes, including soldiers dying as a result of sanitary defects in their

Nightingale's health campaigns, augmenting her own personal political influence, which she reckoned was equivalent to two members of parliament.

barracks in peacetime, impoverished sick people in workhouses, British women in childbirth, the health of indigenous peoples in Australia and New Zealand, and the health of children in the schools of the British empire.) As a health campaigner, Nightingale influenced politicians and administrators one-on-one, using facts and persuasion. As the quote shows, she could also appeal over the heads of politicians to the general public, shaming the government for its lack of care or attention to the health of ordinary poor people. Her main causes in India were to improve the supply of clean water and the provision of sanitation, health education, and measures to prevent famines.

The final two quotes are from her extensive body of writings on leadership directed at nurses. Nightingale found leadership lessons from observing animals and from world religions, mythology, history, and current affairs, but particularly from the Bible. Although the Nightingale Training School for Nurses—which she established in 1860—was secular, the moral tone was Christian, and it is clear from her formal letters that she herself was inspired by stories of heroism and self-sacrifice that she recounted to the nurses during their training. Her leadership model could be described as being based on a vision of health care improvement, with nurses having a sense of their own purpose, exercising authority based on their moral characters, and being members of a mutually supportive profession.

Nightingale communicated about leadership at all levels: to the public through her *Notes on Nursing*, to nurses in training through yearly formal letters, and through the mentoring of chosen nurse leaders. If the question is asked who her followers were, the group is much wider, with many members of European royal families and politicians—figures such as Henri Dunant and Mahatma Gandhi. Such is Nightingale's fame and continuing influence that there is a danger of ascribing too much to her as the founder of modern nursing. An important distinction needs to be drawn on the one hand, between what Nightingale actually said and did and the rather less instructive saintly glow, which she attracted during the Crimean War.

reflective practice

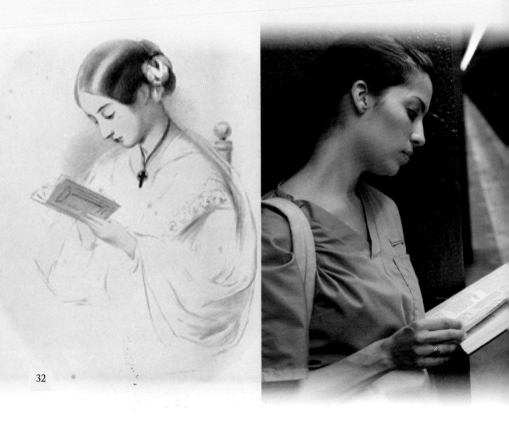

"I desire for a considerable time only to lead a life of obscurity and toil, for the purpose of allowing whatever I may have received of God to ripen, and turning it some day to the glory of His Name. Nowadays people are too much in a hurry both to produce and consume themselves. It is only in retirement, in silence, in meditation, that are formed the men who are called to exercise an influence on society." (Undated note on the writings of Lacordaire, the French Dominican priest)

taking action

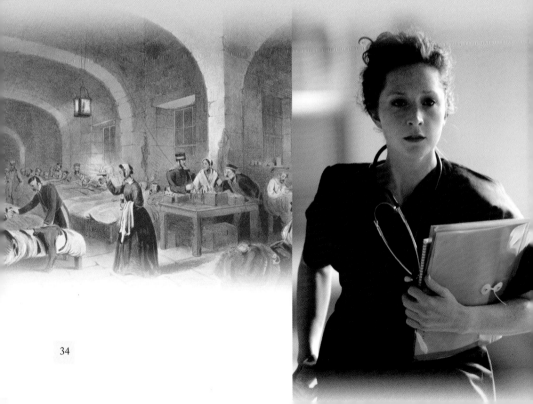

"*I have had a larger responsibility of human lives than ever man or woman had before. And I attribute my success to this: I never gave or took an excuse. Yes, I do see the difference now between me and other men. When a disaster happens, I act and they make excuses.*"

(Letter to Hilary Bonham Carter, 1861)

exercising leadership

"We do not care for the people of India. This is a very heavy indictment. But how else account for the facts about to be given? We even do not care enough to know about their daily lives of lingering death from causes which we could so well remove."

(Opening lines of an article in The Nineteenth Century, 1878)

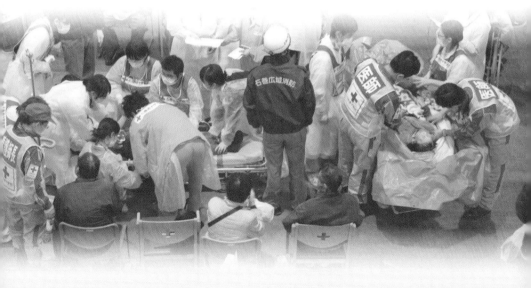

leadership lessons

"To be 'in charge' is certainly not only to carry out the proper measures yourself but to see that everyone else does so too; to see that no one either willfully or ignorantly thwarts or prevents such measures. It is neither to do everything yourself, nor to appoint a number of people to each duty, but to ensure that each does that duty to which he is appointed. This is the meaning which must be attached to the word by (above all) those 'in charge' of sick, whether of numbers or of individuals."
(Notes on Nursing, 2nd edition, 1860)

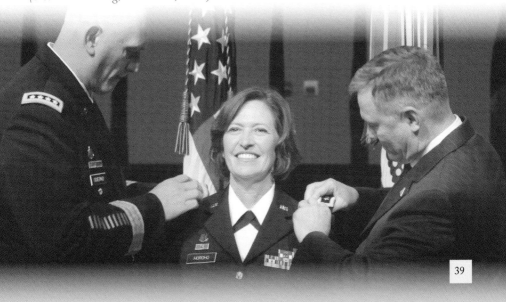

39

your own purpose

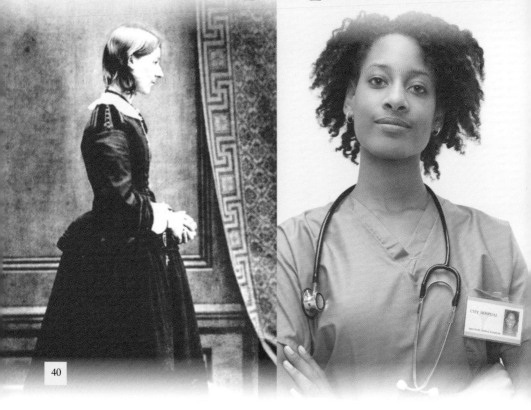

"The very first element for having control over others, is, of course, to have control over oneself. If I cannot take charge of myself, I cannot take charge of others. The next, perhaps, is—not to try to 'seem' anything, but to be what we would seem. A person in charge must be felt more than she is heard—not heard more than she is felt. She must fulfill her charge without noisy disputes, by the silent power of a consistent life, in which there is no seeming, and no hiding, but plenty of discretion. She must exercise authority without appearing to exercise it. A person … in charge must have a quieter and more impartial mind than those under her, in order to influence them by the best part of them and not by the worst."

(First formal letter to the nurses, 1872)

theory

Photograph of Florence Nightingale with probationer nurses from the Nightingale Training School for Nurses at St. Thomas' Hospital in 1886. The probationers and nurses from her school were the recipients of her

There is a timeless sense to the nursing quotes selected here, and they represent Florence Nightingale's most important contribution to thinking on nursing: the definition of holistic patient care, which acknowledges the multifaceted needs of the patient. The hallmarks of her writings are wisdom and common sense in the care of patients and the management of the sick room. The role of the nurse was essentially to make alterations to the environment in terms of fresh air, light, warmth, cleanliness, and quiet; also, she was to select and administer diet "at the least expense of vital power to the patient."

After the publication of the first edition of *Notes on Nursing: What It Is, and What It Is Not*, Florence Nightingale wrote two other editions. The longer second edition, aimed at professional nurses, includes many details of nursing practice that have not endured as well as the first edition—for example, the advice on pulse taking in diagnosis. The third, the shortest edition of the three, is a public health text targeted at the "laboring classes," with its additional chapter on "Minding Baby."

formal letters and, in later years, she followed their careers and gave encouragement to a great many nurses.

The very timelessness and success of the first edition raised a challenge: Did Nightingale intend nursing knowledge to be universal and unchanging? Is progress in nursing moving us away from Nightingale's universal principles? This is in fact a false debate. Nightingale recognized the value of both, as can be demonstrated from Nightingale's writings on nursing after her *Notes on Nursing*.

Although she never completely rewrote *Notes on Nursing*, a close study of articles and letters written by her over the ensuing 40 years shows clearly that she understood and valued progress in nursing, a fact some historians have cast doubt on. One of her reasons for encouraging continuing learning in her formal letters to nurses was the recognition that every 5-10 year period "really requires a second [nurse] training nowadays." In 1893, she wrote: "We are only on the threshold of nursing. In the future, which I will not see, for I am old, may a better way be opened!"

If Florence Nightingale had brought *Notes on Nursing* up to date, she might have included the germ theory, which had huge ramifications for the practice of nursing in the latter part of the 19th century. By 1882, she was giving nurses advice on how to kill germs by washing hands with chlorinated soda. Right at the end of her years of active involvement with the Nightingale Training School, a new revolution appeared in the form of aseptic technique, which she summarized with characteristic wit as "boiling yourself . . . & everything within your reach, including the Surgeon."

The final quote selected demonstrates another subtle development in Nightingale's thinking: She softened her previous authoritarian tone, which she had always justified in the context of the sick room, in recognition that firmness and decisiveness were characteristics that the nurse could deploy to save patients from making energy-wasting decisions over their care. Nightingale recognized that in the context of health promotion—or health nursing, which loomed large in her writings of the 1890s—a more equal partnership between nurse and patient was key to successful communication.

The study of Nightingale's writings on nursing is highly rewarding, not just because of the timelessness of some core aspects concerned with the centrality of patients and their needs, but to see the importance of the continuing development of nursing thought. After all, we too live in a changing world, and as my experience at the Florence Nightingale Museum taught me, nurses of different generations have much to learn from each other.

environment

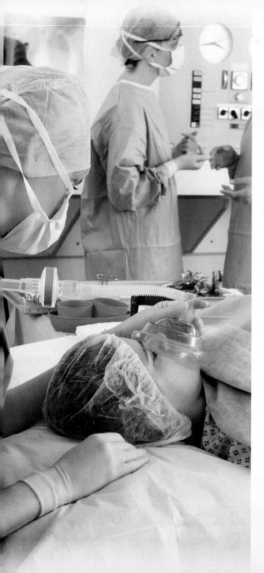

"*Unnecessary noise, or noise that creates an expectation in the mind, is that which hurts a patient. It is rarely the loudness of the noise, the effect upon the organ of the ear itself which appears to affect the sick. How well a patient will generally bear, e.g., the putting up of a scaffolding close to the house, when he cannot bear the talking still less the whispering, especially if it be of a familiar voice, outside his door.*" (Notes on Nursing, 1860)

47

be accountable

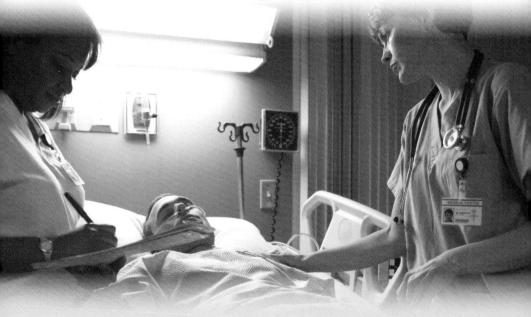

"If a patient is cold, if a patient is feverish, if a patient is faint, if he is sick after taking food, if he has a bed-sore, it is generally the fault not of the disease, but of the nursing." *(Notes on Nursing, 1860)*

49

patient needs

"Every careful observer of the sick will agree in this that thousands of patients are annually starved in the midst of plenty, from want of attention to the ways which alone make it possible for them to take food." (Notes on Nursing, 1860)

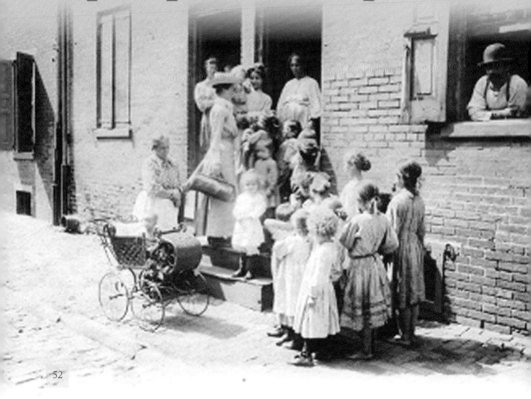

equal partnership

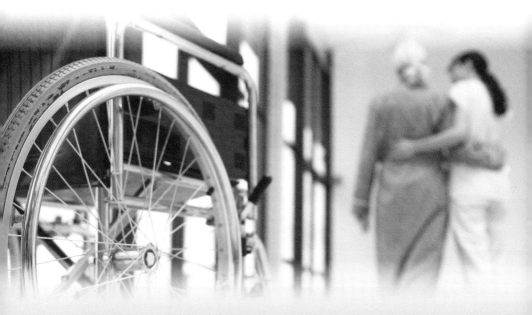

"*We must not talk to them or at them but with them.*"

(Rural Hygiene, 1894)

mind and body

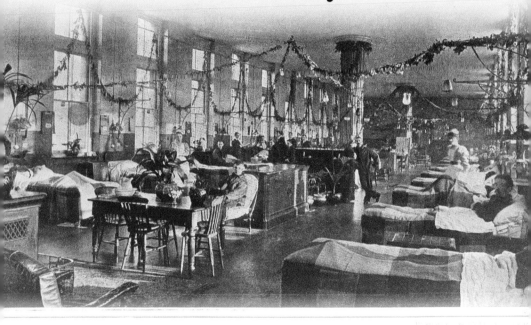

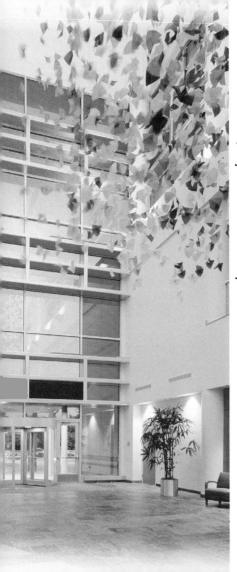

"The effect in sickness of beautiful objects, of variety of objects, and especially of brilliancy of color, is hardly at all appreciated … I have seen, in fevers (and felt, when I was a fever patient myself), the most acute suffering produced from the patient … not being able to see out of window. … People say the effect is only on the mind. It is no such thing. The effect is on the body, too. Little as we know about the way in which we are affected by form, by color, and light we do know this, that they have an actual physical effect. Variety of form and brilliancy of color in the objects presented to patients are actual means of recovery." *(Notes on Nursing, 1860)*

55

legacy

Photograph of Florence Nightingale in bed in her home on South Street in London, taken by her housekeeper, Elizabeth Bosanquet, in 1906. While researching her biography on Florence Nightingale in the mid–1990s,

Florence Nightingale's working methods are interesting and enlightening. She continually sought to direct and refine the focus of her legacy, which sprang from her early vision and was shaped by her opportunities and experiences. One of the benefits of such clarity was that it made it easier to draw a line with public inquiries. She did not give away her precious time unless her correspondents were offering to further her causes. She left behind a large collection of approximately 15,000 letters and other manuscripts, and nearly 200 printed writings, many of which are available today online or in new reprints. The extensiveness of the archive, and her legacy itself, is a reflection of Florence Nightingale's self-discipline, focus, and ruthless time management.

One of my favorite stories from Florence Nightingale's later life is about when she was asked to lend her "relics" for display in a great exhibition. She refused to lend her portrait as a "relic" of the Crimean War because she wanted to discourage hero worship. Instead, she told the organizer off, telling her what the real relics were. The first quote shows Nightingale deflecting personal attention toward her real legacy to the health of the army, trained

holistic nurse and author Barbara Dossey met Sibella Bonham Carter, who had sat on Nightingale's bed at South Street as a small child. Nightingale's legacy lives through such personal links, as well as through history.

nursing, and hygiene. As a result of the feelings expressed in the letter quoted here, she managed to have her bust displayed in the section of modern nursing of Queen Victoria's Diamond Jubilee Exhibition.

A similar episode took place a few years before when Thomas Edison asked her, through a representative, to record her voice on his newly invented wax cylinder phonograph. It is hard for us to appreciate this crackly recording as new technology, but it was one of the wonders of the age, and Nightingale is immortalized putting forward her legacy: "the great work of my life." The British Library holds an original recording that can be listened to on the Internet. Mark Bostridge, a recent biographer of Nightingale, quotes the response to hearing it from the political diarist Harold Nicolson: "She says the last words as if she was signing her signature on a check. 'Florence' (pause) 'Nightingale' (defiantly)." The recording brings to mind the importance of conducting oral history. Many nurses participate in significant innovations in their practice that deserve to be recorded. It is part of our responsibility to the future to ensure that today's achievements are documented for posterity.

The third and fourth quotes summarize an attitude that was clear in Nightingale's final writings. Great as her own contributions had been to nursing and health reform across the world, she was keen for her own generation's work to be surpassed in the interest of progress in saving lives.

In her formal letter to the nurses of 1883, Nightingale advised her nurses to rejoice in the successes of others as if they were their own (see page 76). She followed her own advice, and it is an interesting fact that the first major biography of Florence Nightingale concluded with her own words, reproduced in the final quote, which were from Nightingale's eulogy to Robert Loyd-Lindsay, a Crimean veteran and founder of the British Red Cross.

lessons from war

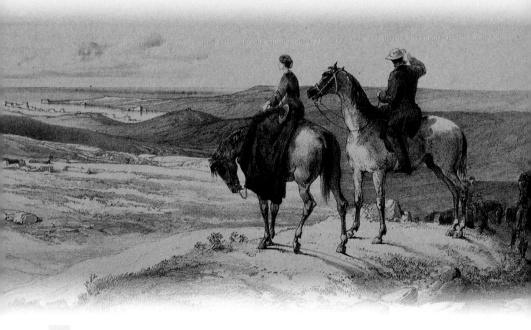

"The 'relics,' the 'representations' of the Crimean War! What are they? They are, first, the tremendous lessons we have had to learn from its tremendous blunders and ignorances. And next they are Trained Nurses and the progress of Hygiene. These are the 'representations' of the Crimean War. And I will not give my foolish portrait (which I have not got) or anything else as 'relics' of the Crimea. It is too ridiculous. You don't judge even the victuals inside a public-house by the sign outside. I won't be made a sign at an exhibition." *(Letter, 1897)*

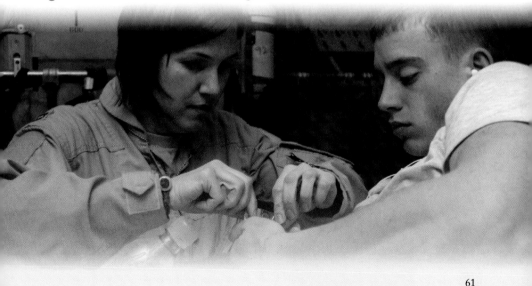

her voice

(Phonograph recording, 1890.
http://www.youtube.com/watch?v=ax3B4gRQNU4)

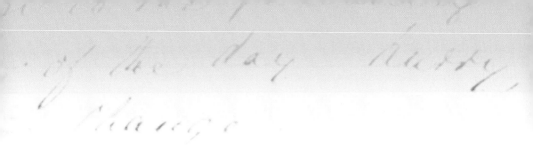

"When I am no longer even a memory, just a name, I hope my voice may perpetuate the great work of my life. God bless my dear old comrades of Balaclava and bring them safe to shore. Florence Nightingale."

progression

"'No system can endure that does not march.' Are we walking to the future or to the past? Are we progressing or are we stereotyping? We remember that we have scarcely crossed the threshold of uncivilized civilization in nursing: there is still so much to do. Don't let us stereotype mediocrity." *(Sick Nursing and Health Nursing, 1893)*

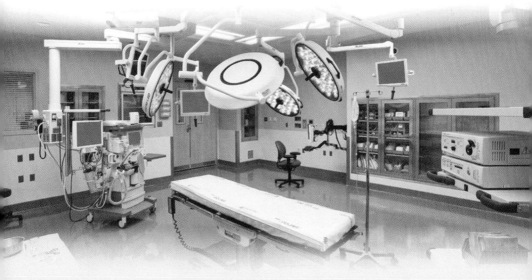

the future

"In the future, which I will not see, for I am old, may a better way be opened! May the methods by which every infant, every human being, will have the best chance of health—methods by which every sick person will have the best chance of recovery, be learned and practiced! Hospitals are only an intermediate stage of civilization, never intended, at all events to take in the whole sick population." (Sick Nursing and Health Nursing, 1893)

make a difference

"One whose life makes a great difference for all:
All are better off than if he had not lived."
(Letter, 1901)

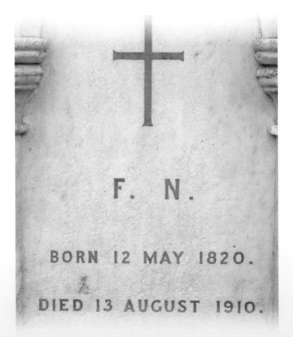

From

Florence Nightingale

to the

Probationer-Nurses

in the

"Nightingale Fund" Training School,

at

St Thomas's Hospital,

and to the

Nurses who were formerly trained there.

23rd May, 1883.

23 May, 1883
My very dear friends
Here is my love with all my heart.
I hope to make the acquaintance of every one of you.
And that will be better even
than being one of you today in body. I am
with you in spirit. That is nothing new.
That is always, always – the old, old story.
And it is the old, old question too: Are we
all of us on our mettle in our life's work?
Joy to us if we are. If not,
there can only be disappointment.

To those of us in earnest in our desire to be
thorough workers – thorough
women – thorough Nurses – (and no woman
can be a good Nurse unless she is a good
woman). We say watch & persevere to do
well your appointed work to fill thoroughly
your present place: don't give in to the
prevailing spirit of the day: hurry,
bustle, change.
To those of us who are halfhearted (I do not
know any but there may be such) we say

71

pause, either turn over a new leaf
or give up the work altogether for if
we remain halfhearted,
(& no one can do the work,
unless she put her whole heart in it)
we are taking up the room of better
women, better workers. The eyes of
England & perhaps of a still
farther & larger world are upon us
to pick out our inconsistencies and
short comings.
Many sneering remarks are made
unworthy of notice. But
(let this old woman whisper, just between ourselves:
I have got my profit all my life out
of sneering remarks)
is there not some foundation for the
epithets, "conceited Nightingales,"
etc., etc., etc.?

What is training? We can't put into
you what is not there. We want to bring
out what is there. Training is enabling
you to use the means you have in

yourselves. Training is drawing out
what you know yourselves. Learn your
work thoroughly in your year
of training. Store it up & practice
it in your brain, eyes & hands, so that you may
always know where to find it, & these – brain,
eyes & hands – may always be
your ready servants.

But don't depend on – don't stop at your year's
training. If you don't go on, you
will fall back. Aim higher. In the second year
& the third year & all your lives,
you will have to train yourselves
on the foundation you have had in your first.
And – you will find, if you are a true Nurse,
you have only just begun.
But – when you have put your hand to
the plough, don't look back.

We here below cannot judge the motives
which bring you into the work.
Let us all have the benefits of the

opinion that some high resolve or
pure motive actuated us.
But how when we become Nurses
do we keep that high resolve, that pure
motive ever in view? – Are we proud to
be Nurses? – to be called Nurse? –
not simply to take pride in dressings & work
which will bring us notice & praise?
Remember, the Nurse is wanted most
by the most helpless & often
most disagreeable cases, in one
sense there is no credit in nursing
pleasant patients.
And don't despise what some of you
call "housemaid's work." If you thought of
its extreme importance, you
would not mind doing it.
As you know, without thorough housemaid's
work, every thing in the Ward or sick room
becomes permeated with organic matter.
The greatest compliment I ever
thought I, as a Hospital Nurse,
received was that I was put to clean &
"do" the Special Ward, with
the severest medical or surgical case

*which I was nursing, every day because I
did it thoroughly & without
disturbing the Patient. That was
the first Hospital I ever served in
(I think I could give a lesson in hospital
housemaid work now).
We Nurses should remember to help
out suffering fellow creatures
in our calling – not to amuse
ourselves, let us make our "calling" "sure."
Sisters, Nurses, Probationers shall we start afresh?
Shall we all renew – as we every
morning need to do – our resolve?
As a friend, a Nurse, abroad said to me:
one must be converted not once but
every day. Shall it be our aim to be
more thorough workers, more
thorough women, more thorough
Nurses every day, till we
become most thorough, & so
live down any spiteful sneers & epithets?
One word nurses: Year by
year our numbers increase.*

We are becoming a large band.
See that we are banded together by
mutual good will and remember the conduct
of each member reflects credit or
discredit on the whole. We cannot
isolate ourselves if we would.
Thank God there are numerous other Training Schools
now in existence. Let us give them the
right hand of fellowship. Wherever we
see thorough work, let us feel
those are our sisters.
Let us run the race where all may win:
rejoicing in their successes, as our own, & mourning
their failures, wherever they are,
as our own. We are all one Nurse.
But see that we fall not off.
We must fight the good fight steadily,
with all our heart & all our mind & all our
strength or they may beat us.
And that they will do if we do not hold to our
colours to be true workers, true women, true Nurses.

We are volunteers. Don't let us forget that.
We have chosen our path. Don't
let us be worse soldiers in God's
army than those who are enlisted
or compulsory conscripts.
For the first time for 25 years,
I went out last winter to see the return
of a Regiment of foot from Egypt.
(And we have Nurses too who
volunteered for Egypt & two of them
still are there,
working hard. They all worked hard & well.)
Anybody might have been
proud of these men's appearances – shabby skeletons
they were, campaigning uniform worn out
but well cleaned. Not spruce
or smart or showy, but
alert, silent, steady in discipline
and not a man of them as I am sure,
but thought he had nothing to be
proud of in what he had done, tho' we
might well be proud of them

Now, we don't say Volunteer
take example by this. Assuredly we will be
their true comrades in faithfulness to
reality & duty. It is the same spirit:
the spirit of the nation. Let us stick to it.
The great Duke of Willington said
"all for duty & nothing for reward."

So may all we volunteers & Nurses,
tho' different in many things, be fellows
in duty so may we raise the
standard, higher & higher, of thoroughness –
(& with thoroughness always goes
humility) – of steady, patient,
silent, cheerful work. So may we all be
on the alert – always on our mettle.
Let us be always in the van of wise & noiseless
high training & progress.

God bless you all.
Florence Nightingale
May 23/83

Table of Images

Page #	Image Credit	Note
20	Bioderm (www.bioderm.us).	Inset: Expected Total Costs Attributable to Hospital Acquired Infections calculated from TMIT-APIC Healthcare Associated Infections Cost Calculator.
22	The Elmer Belt Florence Nightingale Collection, UCLA.	The cover image of Nightingale's "Mortality of the British Army, at Home and Abroad, and During the Russian War, as Compared with the Mortality of the Civilian Population in England," published in 1858.
23	The Future of Nursing Campaign for Action (www.thefutureofnursing.org)	Cover Page for the Institute of Medicine's *Future of Nursing: Leading Change, Advancing Health* report, 2011.
24	Florence Nightingale Museum, London, UK/The Bridgeman Art Library. FNM321936	First page of the "Register of nurses sent to military hospitals in the East"
25	U.S. Department of Health and Human Services Health Resources and Services Administration	Distribution of the registered nurse population by highest nursing or nursing-related educational preparation, 1980-2008. From the IOM Report on the *Future of Nursing: Leading Change, Advancing Health*.
26	Cornell University Library.	Nightingale's Design for a Pavilion Hospital from *Notes on Hospitals*, third edition, 1863.
26	HDR Architecture.	Blueprint of patient room using evidence for best design practices.
28	Florence Nightingale Museum, London, UK/The Bridgeman Art Library. FNM321949	Photograph of Florence Nightingale in the Blue Room at Claydon House, 1891.
32	Florence Nightingale Museum, London, UK/The Bridgeman Art Library. FNM321929	Color lithograph of Florence Nightingale by Hilary Bonham-Carter, 1854.
32	Thinkstock.com, 86505667	
34	Greater London Council, UK/The Bridgeman Art Library. BAL5603	Sketch of the Barrack Hospital, Scutari, c. 1855, by J.A. Benwell .
34	Thinkstock.com, 111882680	
36	Wikipedia Commons.	Engraving titled "The last of the herd," from *The Graphic*, 6 October 1877, about the plight of animals as well as humans during the great famine in India, 1876-78.

Page #	Image Credit	Note
37	International Federation of Red Cross and Red Crescent Societies. Toshirharu Kato, Japanese Red Cross (p-JPN0065 from http://www.flickr.com/photos/ifrc/).	Nurses and other volunteers from Japan's Red Cross help victims of the 11 March 2011 tsunami that struck Japan.
38	National Army Museum, London/The Bridgeman Art Library. NAM254179	Florence Nightingale visiting the hut hospitals at Balaclava in the Crimean War, *Illustrated London News*.
39	U.S. Army personnel. Courtesy of Rob McIlvainc.	Chief of Staff of the Army Gen. Raymond T. Odierno and Retired Col. Ray Horoho pin three-star epaulets on the shoulders of Lt. Gen. Patricia D. Horoho, the 43rd surgeon general and commanding general of the U.S. Army Medical Command, at a ceremony at Joint Base Myer-Henderson Hall, Virginia, 7 December 2011. Horoho is the first nurse and first woman to be nominated for the position and confirmed by Congress.
40	Photostock.com. 86492459	
40	Sir Edmund Verney, Claydon House	Photograph of Florence Nightingale in 1856
42	Wellcome Library, London. L0010473	Florence Nightingale and Sir Harry Verney with group of nurses at Claydon House.
46	Wellcome Library, London. V0006576	Colour lithograph of a Crimean hospital scene "Women's Mission" by J.A. Vinter.
47	Thinkstock.com. 86511007	
48	Florence Nightingale Museum, London, UK/The Bridgeman Art Library. FNM325774	Lithograph of Florence Nightingale during the Crimean War by Wiliam Hatherell from *The Graphic*, 19 November 1904.
49	Thinkstock.com. sb10069454j-001	
50	Wellcome Library, London. L0011962	Florence Nightingale receiving the wounded soldiers in the entrance to the Barrack Hospital at Scutari. Print of Florence Nightingale at Scutari by Samuel Bellin, after Jerry Barrett, 1861.
51	Thinkstock.com, 120677029	
52	Visiting Nurse Society of Philadelphia.	Photograph of a visiting nurse surrounded by children and adults entering a row house in Philadelphia, c. 1890.

Page #	Image Credit	Note
53	Thinkstock.com, skd239623sdc	
54	Wellcome Library, London. L0014151	Photograph of a Nightingale-style pavilion ward at St. Thomas' Hospital, London, decorated for the holidays, by A. Rischgitz.
55	Mark Ballogg, Steinkamp/Ballogg, Chicago.	Lobby at The Wisconsin Heart Hospital, Wauwatosa.
56	Florence Nightingale Museum, London, UK/The Bridgeman Art Library. FNM 321947	Photograph of Florence Nightingale in bed in her home at South Street in London by her housekeeper Elizabeth Bosanquet, 1906.
60	Wellcome Library, London. V0015438	Florence Nightingale and Mr. Bracebridge at Cathcart's Hill burial ground overlooking the besieged city of Sevastopol.
61	U.S. Air Force photo/Senior Airman Erik Cardenas.	Flight nurse treating soldier in aircraft.
62	Wikipedia Commons	Wax cylinder phonograph
64	Florence Nightingale Museum, London, UK/The Bridgeman Art Library. FNM325770	The North Theatre, St. Thomas' Hospital, London, 1908.
65	www.balloggphoto.com.	Surgery suite at Advocate Good Samaritan Hospital in Downers Grove, Illinois.
66	Florence Nightingale Museum, London, UK/The Bridgeman Art Library. FNM 325775	Sketch of Florence Nightingale in 1907 by Frances de Biden Footner.
66	Mercy Ships (www.mercyships.org)	Dan Bergman, a nurse with Mercy Ships, a fleet of mission-based hospital ships, assists a young patient aboard Mercy Africa.
68	Jan Sutton (http://www.flickr.com/photos/all_things_nautical/)	Florence Nightingale is buried in the family plot at the Church of St. Margaret in East Wellow, Hampshire, very near the family estate of Embley Park.
69	Jan Sutton (http://www.flickr.com/photos/all_things_nautical/)	Florence Nightingale left instructions that only her initials and dates be engraved on her gravestone.
70	Wellcome Library, London, UK. M0002395, M0002397, M0002398, M0002399, M0002400, M0002401, M0002402, M0002403, M0002404, M0002405, M0002406, M0002407, M0002408, M0002409.	Letter from Florence Nightingale to the Probationer Nurses in the "Nightingale Fund" Training School at St. Thomas's Hospital and to the nurses who were formerly trained there. Dated and signed 23rd May, 1883.